Can I tell you about Peanut Allergy?

Can I tell you about...?

The "Can I tell you about...?" series offers simple introductions to a range of limiting conditions and other issues that affect our lives. Friendly characters invite readers to learn about their experiences, the challenges they face, and how they would like to be helped and supported. These books serve as excellent starting points for family and classroom discussions.

Other subjects covered in the "Can I tell you about...?" series

ADHD

Adoption

Anxiety

Asperger Syndrome

Asthma

Autism

Cerebral Palsy

Dementia

Depression

Diabetes (Type 1)

Dyslexia

Dyspraxia

Eating Disorders

Eczema

Epilepsy

ME/Chronic Fatigue Syndrome

OCD

Parkinson's Disease

Pathological Demand Avoidance Syndrome

Selective Mutism

Stammering/Stuttering

Stroke

Tourette Syndrome

Can I tell you about Peanut Allergy?

A guide for friends, family and professionals

SHARON DEMPSEY

Illustrated by Alice Blackstock

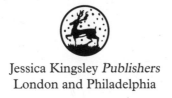

Jessica Kingsley *Publishers*
London and Philadelphia

First published in 2015
by Jessica Kingsley Publishers
73 Collier Street
London N1 9BE, UK
and
400 Market Street, Suite 400
Philadelphia, PA 19106, USA

www.jkp.com

Copyright © Sharon Dempsey 2015
Illustrations copyright © Alice Blackstock 2015

Library of Congress Cataloging in Publication Data
A CIP catalog record for this book is available from the Library of Congress

British Library Cataloguing in Publication Data
A CIP catalogue record for this book is available from the British Library

ISBN 978 1 84905 593 2
eISBN 978 1 78450 067 2

Printed and bound by Bell and Bain Ltd, Glasgow

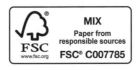

MIX
Paper from
responsible sources
FSC
www.fsc.org
FSC® C007785

Contents

Acknowledgements

Special thanks to the following individuals and organisations who have kindly provided their expertise:

- Dr David M. Edgar BSc (Hons), MB BCh BAO, FRCP (Edin), FRCP (Lond), FRCPath, Consultant Immunologist, The Royal Hospitals, Belfast

- Dr Graham Roberts, Professor and Honorary Consultant Paediatrician in Paediatric Allergy and Respiratory Medicine, Southampton University Hospital NHS Trust

- Professor Jürgen Schwarze, Dr. med., FRCPCH, MRC Centre for Inflammation Research, The University of Edinburgh

- Dr Diab Haddad, Consultant Paediatrician, St Peter's Hospital, Surrey

- Kate Grimshaw, Research Fellow and Dietitian, University of Southampton

- Jamie Kabourek, Resource Manager, Food Allergy Research and Resource Program (FARRP), University of Nebraska–Lincoln

- Mary Alice Cookson, writer

- Lucy Buckroyd (for her editing expertise)

- Irish Food Allergy Network

- British Society for Allergy and Clinical Immunology (BSACI)

Disclaimer

Management of a peanut allergy focuses on teaching parents and children to avoid eating or otherwise coming into contact with peanuts or, in some cases, tree nuts; how to recognise early symptoms of an allergic reaction; and the treatment of symptoms, especially in an emergency situation. It is important to note that each case is individual and what is recommended for one child can be different to another.

While there is much debate within the medical profession about many aspects of nut allergy, this book offers a starting point to discuss the issues with your child and also with health professionals.

This book is for information only and is not intended to replace medical advice. It should not be used for the diagnosis or treatment of a peanut allergy and any questions or concerns should be raised with your health professional.

Introduction

A diagnosis of a peanut allergy can be frightening. Nuts seem to be everywhere, hidden in all sorts of foods, and food labelling does not always help. Most parents respond to the diagnosis by feeling over-protective and by trying to drill the risks into their child in the hope that they avoid nuts at all costs. I understand this; I was one of those parents.

Food allergies often occur in children with a history of asthma, eczema or hay fever. There is an inherited factor in these conditions so there may be a greater risk of developing the condition if they are manifest in family members.

Like many allergies, and other long-term health conditions, understanding is critical to dealing with any problems should they arise. This book aims to explain what a peanut allergy is, how to prevent it and what to do should an emergency arise.

Total avoidance of peanuts, and all products containing peanuts or at risk of cross-contamination by peanuts, is the most effective way of controlling a peanut allergy. Understanding the risks and being able to communicate these risks with friends, family and teachers is the best way of ensuring that your child avoids peanuts.

Being prepared for all emergency situations helps to ensure that, should a reaction occur, you have the correct medicine and procedures in place to deal with it appropriately. Most allergic reactions are mild and can be treated with antihistamine medicine.

Anaphylaxis is a life-threatening allergic reaction but it is rare. Anaphylactic shock is an emergency condition requiring immediate medical attention. Emergency treatment for anaphylaxis consists of an injection of adrenaline or epinephrine, which raises blood pressure, relieves breathing difficulties and reduces swelling. If the adrenaline pen is administered the child needs to be seen by a health professional even if they appear to be responding well.

The fear of having a peanut allergy can be eliminated by awareness and understanding of the condition, which enables you to develop control over the condition. Living well with a peanut allergy is possible with understanding of the condition, vigilance about what foods your child eats and total avoidance of nuts.

I hope this book helps you and your child to understand peanut allergy and to develop effective ways of explaining the condition to others.

It is important to note that there are differences between how a nut allergy and a peanut allergy are managed in different countries. Not all schools adopt a nut or peanut-free policy and not all doctors routinely prescribe adrenaline pens. Not all children who have a peanut allergy will be allergic to all nuts. While peanuts are a different food from tree nuts, studies have shown that there is an increased risk of having an allergy to one or more types of tree nuts (and vice versa).

Furthermore, food labelling may differ between countries and the advice is: if you are in doubt about the ingredients in a food then avoid eating it.

If you have any concerns about the management of your child's condition then discuss it with your medical team. We hope that this book provides a starting point for discussing the issues surrounding a peanut allergy and that it helps your child understand the condition and feel better prepared in explaining it to others.

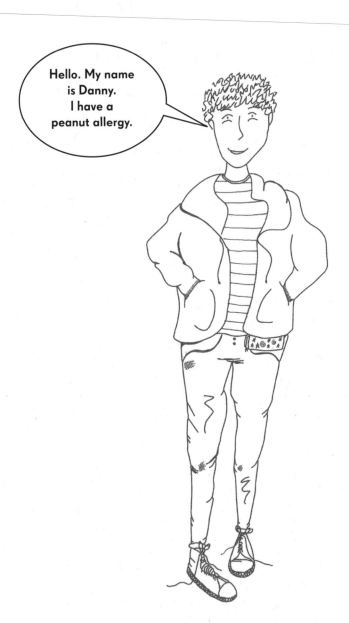

"Hello. My name is Danny. I
have a peanut allergy."

"I am going to tell you about my peanut allergy, what it means and how I manage it. I hope this will help you understand my allergy and how you can help me.

I was diagnosed with a peanut allergy when I was six years old. At first I found it hard to understand that eating peanuts or foods that contain peanuts could be dangerous for me. Peanut allergy means that I cannot eat peanuts and I have to be careful about what I eat in case there are peanuts in it. I am learning to check ingredients and to ask, 'Does this contain peanuts?'

An allergy occurs when the immune system over-reacts to a substance that is harmless to most people. If I eat a peanut my immune system releases antibodies to attack it.

Managing my peanut allergy seemed difficult at first, but now that I understand it better, it isn't so bad.

There is no cure for a peanut allergy but as long as I avoid nuts and foods containing peanut ingredients then I am absolutely fine. It can be difficult eating out in restaurants and going on holiday but usually I can manage my allergy with no problems at all. The important thing to remember is to always check that the food I am eating doesn't contain peanuts and to tell anyone cooking for me that I have a peanut allergy."

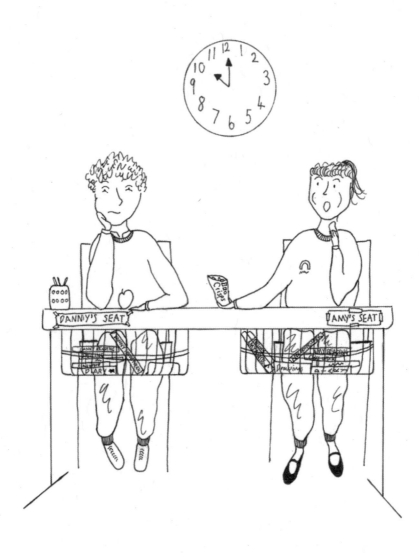

"My allergy means that I have to be careful
not to share food with other people."

"When I was first diagnosed with a peanut allergy I was worried. I didn't want to have to check everything I was going to eat and I certainly didn't want to stop eating certain foods like flapjacks or cookies.

'It is no fun having a food allergy,' I thought, 'especially one which seems to be hidden in lots of nice treats.' I couldn't share snacks with my friends in case they had something with peanuts in it. My friends have been understanding about making sure they do not eat foods containing peanuts when I am around.

Mum said my little sister Lucy could have a peanut allergy too as it is more common in siblings. She is too young to eat peanuts so we don't know yet if she is affected. Gran and Granddad said they wouldn't have peanut products at their house in case I ate something by mistake.

At first my mum was very strict about what I ate. She would panic every time I went to a friend's house and insist on making sure I understood that my allergy is serious. Mum and Dad worry about me eating dinner at my friends' houses or staying over with them. Mum always talks to my friends' parents before I go to their house to make sure they understand about my allergy and she makes sure I have my adrenaline pen (more about that to come) with me at all times."

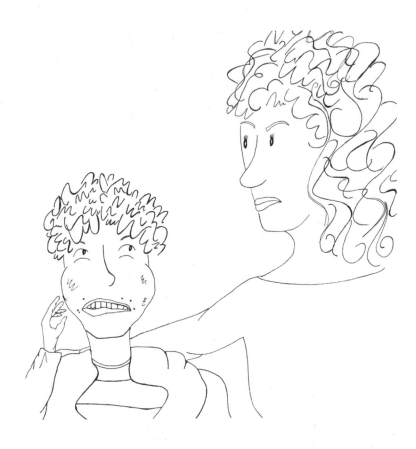

"When I first had a reaction to peanuts my face swelled up and I had a red rash around my mouth. My tongue felt funny and I was frightened."

"Since my diagnosis I have learnt a lot about my allergy and peanuts. For instance, I have discovered that peanuts are actually a legume, not a nut. A legume is a type of plant with seeds that grow inside pods like peas and lentils. Peanuts grow underground, as opposed to nuts like walnuts and almonds that grow on trees.

The proteins in peanuts are similar to those in tree nuts. For this reason, people who are allergic to peanuts can also be allergic to tree nuts, such as almonds, Brazil nuts, walnuts, hazelnuts, macadamias, pistachios, pecans and cashews. I am allergic to peanuts but I avoid all types of nuts just in case.

Mum told me that it is important for me to be aware of how I feel if I do eat peanuts by mistake. Some reactions are mild but others can be very serious. Not everyone has the same allergic reaction. Some people react to peanuts with a rash which looks like hives or nettle stings, or a swelling around the mouth and a scratchy dry feeling in their throat. For others it is a more serious reaction that affects their breathing. It can feel as if there is a tightness in your throat or you can wheeze like having asthma."

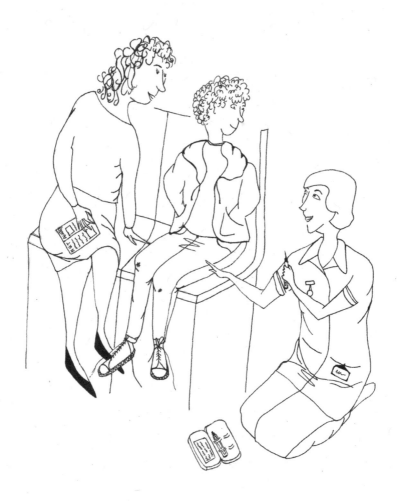

"The adrenaline pen is a special injector pen that injects a dose of adrenaline to treat bad reactions."

"When I was diagnosed Dr Owen explained that I need to always have access to an adrenaline pen (also called epinephrine) and to carry two with me when I am away from home. This is an injecting pen that is used to give me medicine to treat a dangerous allergic reaction in an emergency situation. Along with antihistamine medication, this is part of my emergency medication.

Sometimes antihistamines are used for mild reactions. These might include a rash or swelling, but if I have any difficulty breathing or feel faint, that might mean that I am having a more severe reaction.

The adrenaline pen is an auto-injector pen that injects a dose of adrenaline to treat severe reactions. Mum and Dad had to learn how to use the adrenaline pen for emergencies. I carry two in a little pouch attached to my jacket and make sure they are with me at all times when I am out with friends.

The allergy nurse talked about using the injector pen and told me that I shouldn't worry because if I avoided nuts then I probably wouldn't need it.

A serious reaction is called anaphylaxis (pronounced ANA-FIL-AX-IS). When anaphylaxis occurs the whole body is affected. Usually it means that it's difficult to breathe, or I might feel faint or collapse. This can also be called anaphylactic shock."

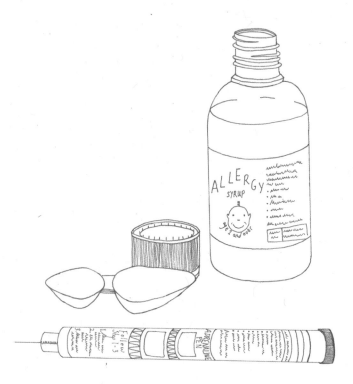

"My antihistamine medicine and my adrenaline pen are used to treat a reaction if I eat peanuts by mistake."

"Once I ate a cookie with peanuts in it – I didn't realise it contained peanuts until it was too late. I struggled to breathe. My throat felt tight and scratchy and my tongue was swollen. I felt faint and scared. Thankfully my mum used the adrenaline pen immediately. I recovered from that reaction but had to go to hospital to be checked out. I am much more careful now.

Touching a peanut can cause a localised reaction. This means that my skin can go red and itchy or a hive-like rash can appear. This wouldn't usually lead to a severe reaction, so if this happened I would take antihistamine medicine.

It is important for me to recognise the signs that I am having a reaction.

Even if I eat peanuts by mistake I can tell by how my body reacts. If it is a mild reaction such as itchy, tingly lips, my tongue feels funny or I develop a rash that looks like hives, then I need to take some antihistamine medicine. Sometimes the reaction can be much more severe and dangerous. My adrenaline pen is used to give me emergency medicine if I am having a bad reaction. If there is any doubt about the severity of a reaction, then it is best to use my adrenaline pen.

Your doctor will discuss what to do in an emergency with you and explain how to use your adrenaline pen. You will also be told about antihistamines, which may be recommended for mild reactions by some doctors."

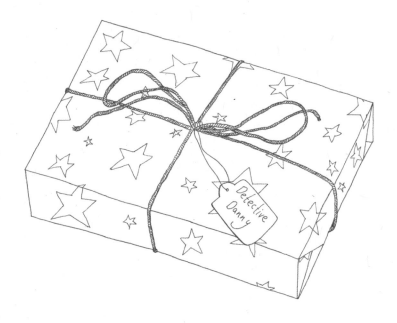

"My mum gave me a magnifying
glass to check the food labelling
ingredients. It is important to check the
ingredients on all the food I eat."

"Not long after I was diagnosed, my birthday was coming up but because of my peanut allergy I didn't feel like having a party.

I didn't want to be worried about everything I ate but Mum explained that if we chose the right foods there would be no problem. Everything at the party would be nut free.

The following week Mum took me shopping for party food. I didn't want to be dragged around the supermarket while Mum shopped and checked all of the ingredients. When we arrived at the supermarket car park, Mum reached into the glove compartment and pulled out a star-covered parcel, tied up with string.

'What is it?' I asked.

'Look and see,' said Mum. I opened the wrapping and took out a magnifying glass.

It felt heavy and made everything look bigger.

'This,' said Mum, 'is the first peanut ingredient detector magnifying glass. With your magnifying glass and a little help from me, you can choose all the food for your party.'

'Being informed about your allergy will enable you to be in control and help you to avoid eating foods containing nuts by accident.'

She explained that peanut allergy is something that I just have to live with and it doesn't have to feel like a problem as long as I take control of what I eat.

'It is not a big issue if we avoid nuts,' Mum said. "

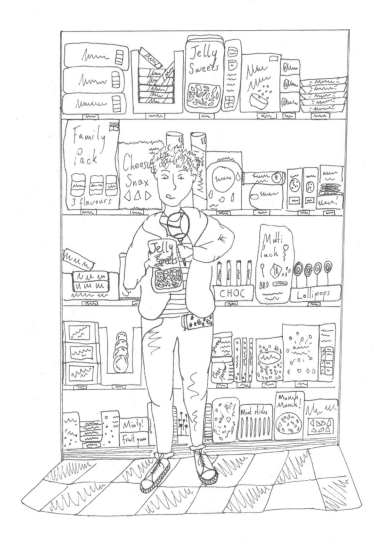

"The ingredient labels can be confusing so I have to check carefully."

"Mum had told me there would be many labels saying 'MADE IN A FACTORY CONTAINING NUTS'. This maddened me because even though the product had no nuts in the ingredients list, I still had to avoid it. The risk was too high.

'Yes!' I said when I found my first party food that stated on the label the magic words, 'MADE IN A NUT-FREE ZONE'.

Mum called me Danny the Peanut Detective because I was so good at spotting the foods I could eat and those that I had to avoid.

I no longer felt angry about my peanut allergy. I understood how important it is to be aware of the ingredients and I realised that with careful checking I could eat lots of different foods and still be safe.

Rules about food labelling are different in each country. Check with your doctor about the guidelines in your country and learn to check and identify which foods are safe to eat.

At the party I was able to explain to my friends what a peanut allergy is and that it is important that they don't give me food that might contain nuts. 'Dr Owen said that even if you just touch my hand while you are eating there is a very small chance that I could still have a mild reaction,' I said. Everyone agreed to make sure we were careful. My friend Sarah's brother also has a peanut allergy so she knew all about what I had to do."

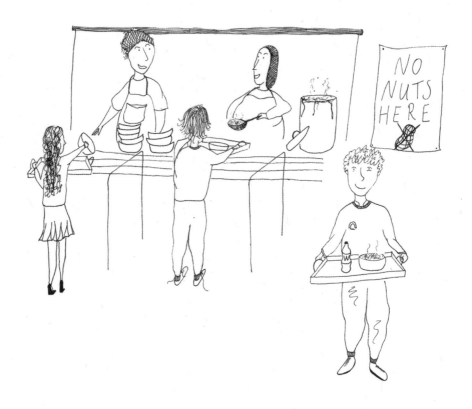

"I like having school dinners with my friends. The canteen always serves nut-free food."

"Mum told my teacher, Mrs Graham, all about my allergy and they discussed how the school could make sure I did not come into contact with peanuts.

The school cafeteria staff are already aware of the dangers of peanut allergy and a poster saying 'NO NUTS HERE' is on the school dining hall wall. Not all schools have a nut-free policy so you might find that your school has a different way of dealing with allergies.

My mum gave the school an Allergy Action Plan sheet, which has details of my allergy and instructions for emergency situations. Mrs Graham has been trained to use the adrenaline pen if I ever need it in an emergency situation.

Most schools are aware of the risks and some, like mine, have a nut-free policy: NO NUTS HERE!

I was happier knowing that everyone understood what a peanut allergy is. Many people told me they knew of someone who had a peanut allergy and I no longer felt alone and like the odd one out.

I know that it is important to tell a teacher straight away if I think I may have eaten peanuts or something containing nuts. If I don't think I have eaten anything with nuts in it but feel unwell and have any of the symptoms of my allergy it is still important that I tell my teacher just in case. A reaction usually occurs within minutes of eating the nuts but sometimes it can be later."

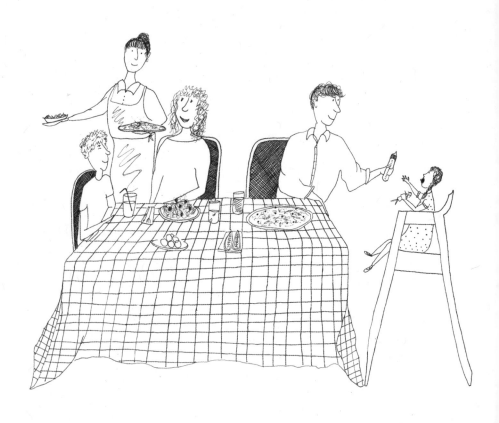

"Having a nut allergy doesn't stop me eating in restaurants. I just have to be careful when I order my food."

"One thing that still worried me was eating out. I love going out to restaurants with my family and I was afraid that I could no longer eat in my favourite restaurant.

Dr Owen advised us that when eating out at restaurants it was best to call ahead and ask if they are able to prepare nut-free dishes.

On Saturday we all went out for pizza. Mum had explained my peanut allergy when she booked the table and when we arrived she asked to speak to the person in charge and explained that I have a peanut allergy and asked for advice on what to order. The restaurant manager made sure the kitchen staff and the waitresses knew about my peanut allergy to avoid cross-contamination – this means my food coming into contact with other food which may have nuts in it. Our waitress was really helpful and wrote 'NUT FREE' on the top of our order just to make doubly sure that everyone dealing with our order knew.

She recommended several dishes that were nut- and peanut-free and I was able to pick my favourites – dough balls, French fries and Margherita pizza followed by chocolate fudge cake. Yummy!

It is very important to be safe and not take any risks.

As Dad said, it was just a matter of checking ingredients and being careful about what I ate."

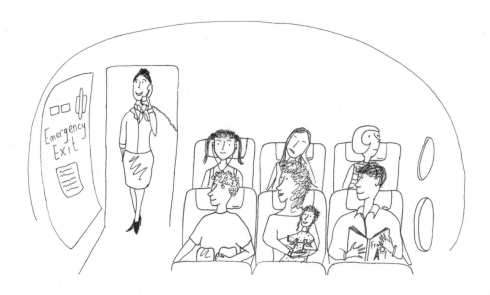

"I was excited to be on the aeroplane
going to France. We had told the airline
all about my allergy in advance."

"Mum and Dad did some research about travelling with a peanut allergy. We discovered that most airlines do not serve nut snacks if you alert them to your peanut allergy in advance. If other passengers on a plane are eating peanuts, there is a small possibility that the dust from the peanuts can cause me problems by circulating in the air in the enclosed environment.

Mum and Dad told our holiday insurers that I have a peanut allergy in case we needed to access hospital care while on holiday. They advised us to carry a letter from our GP explaining the condition and saying that I would be travelling with my adrenaline pens and antihistamine medicine. Mum made sure we carried the adrenaline pens in our hand (carry-on) luggage in case I had a reaction on the plane or in case our luggage was lost!

We decided to book a self-catering apartment in France so that we could prepare my food, as we had to be extra cautious about what I ate.

Our trip to France was fantastic. On the flight the air steward announced that they would not be serving any nut products as they had a nut allergy sufferer on board. *That was me!*

We visited lots of old castles and spent many days on the beach, playing on the sand and swimming in the sea. I made sure that we carried my antihistamine medicine and adrenaline pens everywhere we went and Mum packed plenty of safe snacks for me when we went out and about."

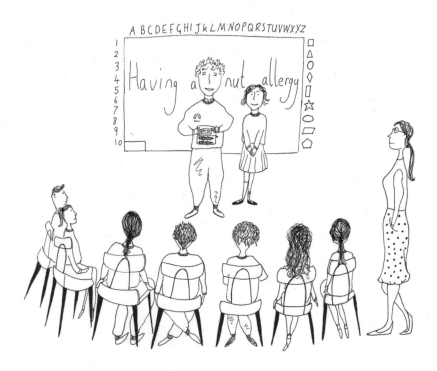

"I can talk to my friends and teachers about my peanut allergy and how it affects me."

"I have had my peanut allergy for two years now and I am able to manage it. The important thing is to be aware of the risks and avoid them. I check everything I eat and if I am in any doubt I just don't have it. I never share snacks or lunches with my friends at school. Even if they think it is safe, there may be a risk.

Last week my teacher asked me to give a talk to the junior school on my allergy. A girl called Anna in Year 3 has just been diagnosed with a peanut allergy too. I was able to explain what it is like to be allergic to peanuts. Everyone agreed that having a peanut allergy is not so bad. I explained the importance of always checking food labels and knowing where your food is prepared.

Anna and I are not alone in having a peanut allergy. Many children and young people have it. We understand that the best way to manage our allergy is to be careful, to check labels and never to eat food if you are not certain of the ingredients and where it has been prepared.

It is also important to raise awareness of peanut allergy. I hope you can pass our message along: If you have a peanut allergy, check before you eat!"

Advice for friends on how to help me

- "First of all be aware of giving me any foods containing peanuts or which may have been contaminated by being near to nuts.

- Don't be frightened of inviting me to your home for dinner or to your birthday party as I still want to be included. I just have to be careful about the food I eat and with some planning we can make sure the food you serve is safe for me.

- Please listen to me and be aware if you think I may be having a reaction to something I may have eaten. If you think I am looking red, flushed, swollen or I am having trouble breathing please get help and tell an adult straight away. It does not help to wait for the symptoms to pass; sometimes the reaction can become rapidly worse. If I say I don't feel well, or that my tongue feels strange or that I feel like I can't breathe please get an adult to help me.

- Know where my emergency medication is kept and tell an adult who knows how to give it to me. Your quick response and care can make a big difference and in extreme cases could save my life."

Advice on how to help me at school

- "It is essential to have a written allergy management plan. This means that should I suffer a reaction in school everyone concerned with my care knows what to do.

- Be aware of the symptoms of my allergy and if I appear unwell, listen to me. I can usually tell if I am having a reaction. Do not tell me to wait and see if it passes.

- My adrenaline pens should be readily available at all times and regularly checked to ensure they are not out of date. There should be people trained to give me the adrenaline pen medication in an emergency situation. It is also important to check the expiry date on the adrenaline pen to ensure it is still effective.

- Inform the parents of all the children at school and especially those in my class that I have a peanut allergy and that it would be better for me if everyone avoided bringing peanuts and foods containing nuts to school. Not all schools enforce a nut or peanut ban. Some schools believe that such a rule is not enforceable and that it presents risks in that the allergic child is less likely to check food if they feel a ban on nuts is in place.

- Communication about allergy awareness is essential so that everyone understands the risks and works together to eliminate them.

- It helps if everyone close to me washes their hands with soap after eating to remove any possible food allergens."

Advice for parents

- "Most allergic reactions to peanuts and tree nuts are mild and usually result in hives, vomiting or some swelling. Management of a peanut allergy and the reactions resulting from coming into contact with peanuts involves:

  - identifying the cause (peanuts) and avoidance

  - being aware of the symptoms of an allergic reaction

  - knowing what to do in an emergency situation.

- Explain the peanut allergy condition to your child's school, friends and relatives.

- Always carry prescribed adrenaline pens with you and know how to use them. Alert restaurants to the condition and read all food labels.

- Keep asthma well managed."

Advice on eating out and travelling

- "It is best to avoid baked goods, confectionery and take-away food served in markets, as the ingredients are often not labelled.

- Telephone the restaurant in advance to see if they serve nut-free options. Make sure the waiting staff are aware and that they inform the kitchen staff too. Check what your child has been served as mix-ups do occur.

- If you are travelling abroad inform your insurance company about your child's peanut allergy.

- Inform the airline of the peanut allergy and ask if they will be able to ensure a nut-free flight.

- Carry your child's emergency kit as hand luggage. This will require a letter from your doctor."

What to do in an emergency

"Symptoms of an allergic reaction include:

- a red, raised, itchy skin rash like hives

- swelling – particularly of the face; the medical term for this is angioedema

- a runny nose

- itchy, runny or red eyes

- feeling sick and/or vomiting and pains in the tummy.

Additional symptoms that may indicate anaphylaxis include:

- any of the above symptoms

- swelling in your throat and narrowing of your airways, which can cause breathing difficulties and wheezing

- a hoarse voice

- a cough

- a sudden drop in blood pressure, which can make you feel faint and dizzy

- a feeling that something very bad is going to happen

- unconsciousness.

A good, easy guide for spotting the signs of anaphylaxis is ABC:

- **A**irways – coughing, swollen tongue, difficulty swallowing, hoarse voice

- **B**reathing – wheezing, noisy breathing or trouble breathing

- **C**onsciousness – dizziness, floppiness, sleepiness, collapse.

Usually a mild reaction is treated with an antihistamine medicine. Be aware of the warning signs and symptoms and if you suspect that the child is not responding to the antihistamine medication then be prepared to administer the epinephrine auto-injector (adrenaline pen). Advice on when to administer the adrenaline pen can vary from country to country and doctor to doctor. In general there is little harm in giving the adrenaline injection; however, the child will need to be checked out by a hospital doctor straight away.

It is important to be aware of the emergency number to call in the country you are in and to phone the emergency services immediately, telling them that the child is experiencing anaphylaxis. If the child has been given the adrenaline they need to be monitored in hospital."

Understanding food labelling

"Different countries have different labelling guidelines, and in some countries the information will vary from brand to brand. Always check the labels carefully. Look out for these warnings:

- 'may contain nuts' (does not necessarily have nuts but could have been made in a factory with other nut products)

- 'may contain nut traces'

- 'cannot guarantee nut free'

- 'not suitable for nut allergy sufferers'

- 'produced in a facility that also processes nuts'.

The manufacturer's ingredients list must be accurate but they use the 'may contain' wording when there is a chance allergens might have got into the product by accident. For example, if the manufacturer's machinery was used to make a product with nuts and then is used to produce the nut-free product cross-contamination could occur. It is a small risk. There are of course no absolute guarantees so please check with your doctor.

Food labelling can change and just because your child has safely eaten a product previously do not assume it has not been subject to change. If a product has a precautionary statement for your child's allergen, then it should be avoided.

These warnings should always be taken seriously."

Facts and figures

- The number of children with peanut allergies has nearly doubled over a five-year period in Europe and America.[1]

- About 1 in 200 children (0.5%) have a reaction to peanuts by the age of five years.[2]

- In the region of 1 in 70 UK children suffer from peanut allergy; the vast majority (approximately 80%) will have this allergy for life.[3]

- About 50 per cent of children with peanut allergy will also have allergies to other nuts.[4]

- If a child has an allergic reaction to peanuts or nuts they must see their GP and be referred to an NHS allergy clinic for confirmation of the diagnosis.[5]

---

1   Allergy UK. "Peanut and Tree Nut Allergy", available at www.allergyuk.org/peanut-and-tree-nut-allergy/peanut-and-tree-nut-allergy, accessed on 21 January 2015.
2   The Children's Hospital at Westmead, Sydney Children's Hospital. "Peanut allergy and Peanut-free diet fact sheet", available at www.schn.health.nsw.gov.au/files/factsheets/peanut_allergy_and_peanut_free_diet-en.pdf, accessed on 21 January 2015.
3   Leap. "Peanut Allergy – in a Nutshell", available at www.leapstudy.co.uk/peanutallergy.html, accessed on 21 January 2015.
4   Dr. David Edgar. "Nut Allergy: Information for patients and their families", available at www.davidedgar.org/PEANUT_29_11_10.doc, accessed on 21 January 2015.
5   Anaphylaxis Campaign. "Peanut allergy and tree nut allergy – the facts", available at www.anaphylaxis.org.uk/userfiles/files/Peanut%20Allergy%20and%20Tree%20Nut%20Allergy%20Factsheet%202012.pdf, accessed on 21 January 2015.

ADDITIONAL NOTES

- There are different types of injectors available.

- It is important to check expiry dates on all medicines and to carry more than one injector pen in case one should break during usage.

Recommended websites and organisations

UK

Action Against Allergy
Phone: 020 8892 2711
Website: www.actionagainstallergy.co.uk
Email: aaa@actionagainstallergy.freeserve.co.uk

Offers help and support for allergy sufferers, food allergy, intolerance and sensitivity.

Allergy Action
Phone: 01727 855 294
Website: http://allergyaction.org

Allergy Action offers information to help allergic people choose food and travel safely. Provides advice and training in food allergen risk management and news about allergy research and training projects.

Allergy UK
Phone: 01322 619898
Email: info@allergyuk.org
Website: www.allergyuk.org

Provides a dedicated helpline, support network and online forum for those with allergies.

Anaphylaxis Campaign
Email: info@anaphylaxis.org.uk
Website: www.anaphylaxis.org.uk

A UK wide charity providing information for the growing numbers of people at risk from severe allergic reactions and anaphylaxis.

Epipen (Meda Pharmaceuticals)
Website: www.epipen.co.uk

This site has a kids' zone with information, printouts and games.

Food Standards Agency
Phone: 020 7276 8829
Email: helpline@foodstandards.gsi.gov.uk
Website: www.food.gov.uk

For information on UK food labelling see: www.food.gov.uk/science/allergy-intolerance/label#toc-2.

The British Society for Allergy & Clinical Immunology (BSACI)
Phone: 0207 501 3910
Email: info@bsaci.org
Website: www.bsaci.org

For Action Plans for children with a peanut or nut allergy see: www.bsaci.org/about/pag-allergy-action-plans-for-children.

Leap (Learning Early About Peanut Allergy)
Website: www.leapstudy.co.uk

The Leap study is a clinical trial looking at how to prevent a peanut allergy in young children.

Nutmums
Website: www.nutmums.com

Provides information and support for parents of nut allergic children.

Ireland
Anaphylaxis Ireland
Phone: 0818 300 238
Email: info@anaphylaxisireland.ie
Website: www.anaphylaxisireland.ie

Anaphylaxis Ireland aims to raise awareness of anaphylaxis and provide support to people at risk and their families.

Irish Food Allergy Network
Website: http://ifan.ie

The website acts as a guide for professionals working with children and families affected by food allergies.

USA

Allergic Living
Website: http://allergicliving.com

This is a magazine site offering advice, recipes and information on living with allergies. It also has a Canadian magazine.

American Academy of Allergy Asthma and Immunology (AAAAI)
Phone: (414) 272-6071
Email: info@aaaai.org
Website: www.aaaai.org/home.aspx

Membership of more than 6,800 worldwide allergists/immunologists and related professionals.

American College of Allergy, Asthma and Immunology (ACAAI)
Website: www.acaai.org

This is a professional organisation with more than 6,800 members in the United States, Canada and 72 other countries. This membership includes allergist/immunologists, other medical specialists, allied health and related healthcare professionals.

Food Allergy Research and Education (FARE)
Website: www.foodallergy.org

Lots of detailed information on food allergies and tools and resources.

The Peanut Institute
Website: www.peanut-institute.org

This is a non-profit organisation that supports nutrition research and develops educational programs to encourage healthful lifestyles that include peanuts and peanut products.

National Institute of Allergy and Infections Diseases

Website: www.niaid.nih.gov

The National Institute of Allergy and Infectious Diseases (NIAID) conducts and supports basic and applied research to better understand, treat, and ultimately prevent infectious, immunologic, and allergic diseases.

PeanutAllergy.com

Website: www.peanutallergy.com

An online allergy community resource site providing a platform to ask questions and share advice.

SelectWisely

Website: www.selectwisely.com/catalog/Nut_Allergies

SelectWisely has a series of cards in different languages explaining nut allergy and requesting nut-free food. These need to be purchased.

US Food and Drug Administration

Phone: 1-888-INFO-FDA (1-888-463-6332)
Website: www.fda.gov

For information on USA food labelling see: www.fda.gov/food/ guidanceregulation/guidancedocumentsregulatoryinformation/ allergens/ucm106890.htm.

Canada

Air Canada

Website: www.aircanada.com/en/travelinfo/onboard/dining/ nutritional.html

Provides details of the company policies regarding flying with a nut allergy.

Allergy/Asthma Information Association

Website: www.aaia.ca/en/index.htm
Phone: 1-800-611-7011
Email: admin@aaia.ca

Provides information, links and guidelines for dealing with allergies in Canada.

EatRight Ontario

Website: www.eatrightontario.ca

Provides information on nutrition and allergies.

Australia

Allergy and Anaphylaxis Australia (A&AA)

Website: www.allergyfacts.org.au

Phone: +61 1300 728 000

Email: coordinator@allergyfacts.org.au

Aiming to improve the awareness of allergy by sharing current information, education, advocacy, research, guidance and support.

Australasian Society of Clinical Immunology and Allergy

Website: www.allergy.org.au

Working to advance the science and practice of allergy and clinical immunology.

New Zealand

Allergy New Zealand

Website: www.allergy.org.nz

A national charity that provides you with reliable information, education and support so you can manage your or your child's allergy and live an active and healthy lifestyle.

Nutrition Foundation NZ

Website: www.nutritionfoundation.org.nz

Phone: +64 9 489 3417

Email: webenquiry@nutritionfoundation.org.nz

Provides information on food, nutrition and allergies.

Blank for your notes

Blank for your notes

Blank for your notes

Blank for your notes

Blank for your notes